This jou belongs to :

Name:
_____

Address:
_____

Emergency Contact Name/Number:
_____

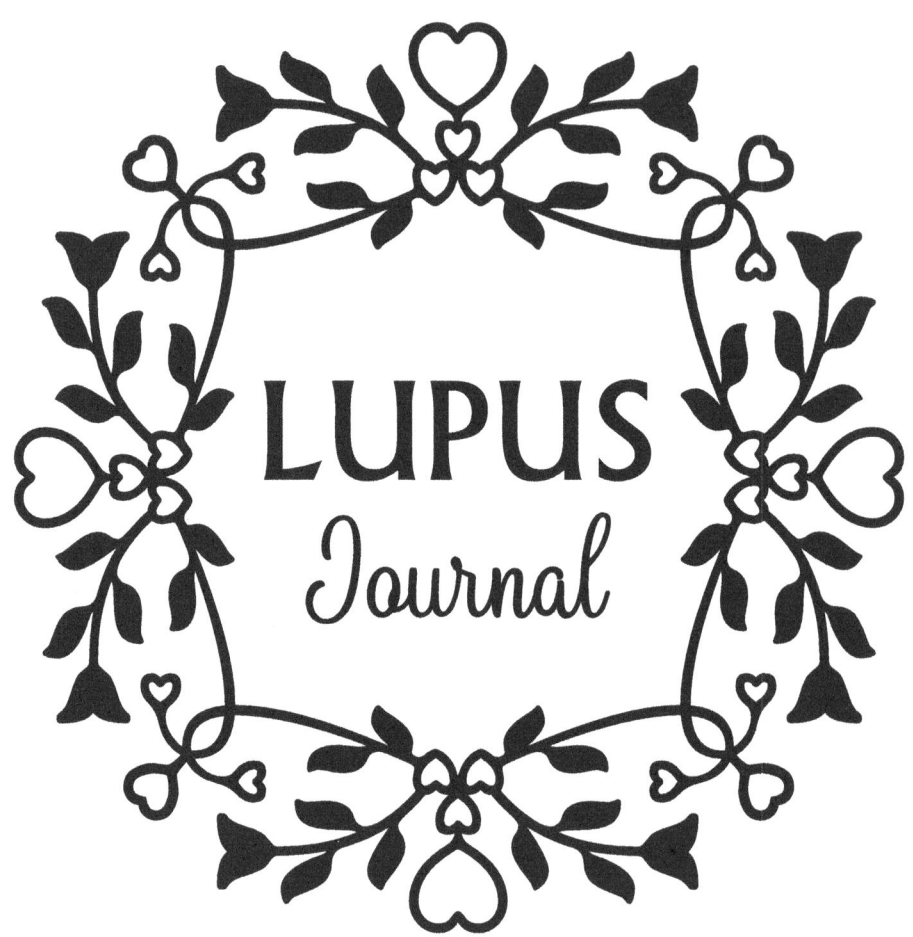

Copyright © Ansart Design
All rights reserved.

For any suggestions or questions regarding our books,
please contact us at: **ansartdesign.contact@gmail.com**

Today's Date: _____

SLEEP _____
_____

BREAKFAST   **LUNCH**   **DINNER**
_____   _____   _____
_____   _____   _____
_____   _____   _____
_____   _____   _____
_____   _____   _____

SNACKS
_____   _____   _____
_____   _____   _____
_____   _____   _____

WATER 🥤 🥤 🥤 🥤 🥤 🥤 🥤 🥤 🥤 🥤 🥤 🥤 🥤
TOTAL: _____

ACTIVITIES
_____
_____
_____
_____

How I feel today about my food

   o 🙂   o 😐   o 🙁

How I feel today about my activities

   o 🙂   o 😐   o 🙁

Mark the pain zones

Front   Right   Back   Left

Time Started:
Time Ended:
Total Duration:

Type of pain: ☐ Tingling
☐ Shooting ☐ Throbbing
☐ Sharp ☐ Aching ☐ Swelling
☐ Burning ☐ Numbness
☐ Cramping ☐ Stiffness ☐ Dull
☐ Other: ─────────

Pain Scale: 1 2 3 4 5 6 7 8 9 10

SYMPTOMS

	PAIN	FATIGUE	ANXIETY	MOOD
AM	/10	/10	/10	/10
PM	/10	/10	/10	/10

TAKEN TODAY

NOTE OF THE DAY

SOMETHING TO MAKE TOMORROW BETTER:

Today's Date : _____

SLEEP _____

BREAKFAST
_____
_____
_____
_____
_____

LUNCH
_____
_____
_____
_____
_____

DINNER
_____
_____
_____
_____
_____

SNACKS
_____
_____
_____

WATER 🥤🥤🥤🥤🥤🥤🥤🥤🥤🥤🥤🥤

TOTAL: _____

ACTIVITIES
_____
_____
_____
_____

How I feel today about my food

○ 🙂   ○ 😐   ○ ☹️

How I feel today about my activities

○ 🙂   ○ 😐   ○ ☹️

Mark the pain zones

Front Right Back Left

Time Started:
Time Ended:
Total Duration:

Type of pain: ☐ Tingling
☐ Shooting ☐ Throbbing
☐ Sharp ☐ Aching ☐ Swelling
☐ Burning ☐ Numbness
☐ Cramping ☐ Stiffness ☐ Dull
☐ Other: _____

Pain Scale: 1 2 3 4 5 6 7 8 9 10

SYMPTOMS

_____ _____ _____
_____ _____ _____
_____ _____ _____

	PAIN	FATIGUE	ANXIETY	MOOD
AM	/10	/10	/10	/10
PM	/10	/10	/10	/10

TAKEN TODAY

_____ _____ _____
_____ _____ _____
_____ _____ _____

NOTE OF THE DAY

_____
_____
_____

SOMETHING TO MAKE TOMORROW BETTER:

_____
_____
_____

Today's Date : _____

SLEEP
_____
_____

BREAKFAST
_____
_____
_____
_____
_____

LUNCH
_____
_____
_____
_____
_____

DINNER
_____
_____
_____
_____
_____

SNACKS
_____
_____
_____

_____
_____
_____

_____
_____
_____

WATER 🥛🥛🥛🥛🥛🥛🥛🥛🥛🥛🥛🥛
TOTAL: _____

ACTIVITIES
_____
_____
_____
_____

How I feel today about my food

○ 🙂   ○ 😐   ○ ☹️

How I feel today about my activities

○ 🙂   ○ 😐   ○ ☹️

Mark the pain zones

Front Right Back Left

Time Started:
Time Ended:
Total Duration:

Type of pain:
- ☐ Tingling
- ☐ Shooting ☐ Throbbing
- ☐ Sharp ☐ Aching ☐ Swelling
- ☐ Burning ☐ Numbness
- ☐ Cramping ☐ Stiffness ☐ Dull
- ☐ Other: _____

Pain Scale: 1 2 3 4 5 6 7 8 9 10

SYMPTOMS

_____ _____ _____
_____ _____ _____
_____ _____ _____

	PAIN	FATIGUE	ANXIETY	MOOD
AM	/10	/10	/10	/10
PM	/10	/10	/10	/10

TAKEN TODAY

_____ _____ _____
_____ _____ _____
_____ _____ _____

NOTE OF THE DAY

_____
_____
_____

SOMETHING TO MAKE TOMORROW BETTER:

_____
_____
_____

Today's Date : _____

SLEEP _____

BREAKFAST	LUNCH	DINNER
_____	_____	_____
_____	_____	_____
_____	_____	_____
_____	_____	_____
_____	_____	_____

SNACKS
_____
_____
_____

WATER 🍺 🍺 🍺 🍺 🍺 🍺 🍺 🍺 🍺 🍺 🍺 🍺

TOTAL: _____

ACTIVITIES
_____
_____
_____
_____

How I feel today about my food

○ 🙂   ○ 😐   ○ ☹️

How I feel today about my activities

○ 🙂   ○ 😐   ○ ☹️

Mark the pain zones

Front   Right   Back   Left

Time Started:
Time Ended:
Total Duration:

Type of pain: ☐ Tingling
☐ Shooting ☐ Throbbing
☐ Sharp ☐ Aching ☐ Swelling
☐ Burning ☐ Numbness
☐ Cramping ☐ Stiffness ☐ Dull
☐ Other: ——————————

Pain Scale: 1 2 3 4 5 6 7 8 9 10

SYMPTOMS

_____ _____ _____
_____ _____ _____
_____ _____ _____

	PAIN	FATIGUE	ANXIETY	MOOD
AM	/10	/10	/10	/10
PM	/10	/10	/10	/10

TAKEN TODAY

_____ _____ _____
_____ _____ _____
_____ _____ _____

NOTE OF THE DAY

_____
_____
_____

SOMETHING TO MAKE TOMORROW BETTER:

_____
_____
_____

Today's Date: _____

SLEEP _____
_____

BREAKFAST   **LUNCH**   **DINNER**
_____   _____   _____
_____   _____   _____
_____   _____   _____
_____   _____   _____

SNACKS
_____   _____   _____
_____   _____   _____

WATER 🥤🥤🥤🥤🥤🥤🥤🥤🥤🥤🥤🥤
                                                    TOTAL: _____

ACTIVITIES
_____
_____
_____
_____

How I feel today about my food

   ○ 🙂   ○ 😐   ○ ☹️

How I feel today about my activities

   ○ 🙂   ○ 😐   ○ ☹️

Mark the pain zones

Front Right Back Left

Time Started:
Time Ended:
Total Duration:

Type of pain: ☐ Tingling
☐ Shooting ☐ Throbbing
☐ Sharp ☐ Aching ☐ Swelling
☐ Burning ☐ Numbness
☐ Cramping ☐ Stiffness ☐ Dul
☐ Other: ─────────

Pain Scale: 1 2 3 4 5 6 7 8 9 10

SYMPTOMS

_____   _____   _____
_____   _____   _____
_____   _____   _____

	PAIN	FATIGUE	ANXIETY	MOOD
AM	/10	/10	/10	/10
PM	/10	/10	/10	/10

TAKEN TODAY

_____   _____   _____
_____   _____   _____
_____   _____   _____

NOTE OF THE DAY

_____
_____
_____

SOMETHING TO MAKE TOMORROW BETTER:

_____
_____
_____

Today's Date: _____

SLEEP _____
_____

BREAKFAST
_____
_____
_____
_____
_____

LUNCH
_____
_____
_____
_____
_____

DINNER
_____
_____
_____
_____
_____

SNACKS
_____
_____
_____

WATER 🍺🍺🍺🍺🍺🍺🍺🍺🍺🍺🍺🍺

TOTAL: _____

ACTIVITIES
_____
_____
_____
_____

How I feel today about my food

○ 🙂   ○ 😐   ○ 🙁

How I feel today about my activities

○ 🙂   ○ 😐   ○ 🙁

Mark the pain zones

Front   Right   Back   Left

Time Started:
Time Ended:
Total Duration:

Type of pain: ☐ Tingling
☐ Shooting   ☐ Throbbing
☐ Sharp   ☐ Aching   ☐ Swelling
☐ Burning   ☐ Numbness
☐ Cramping   ☐ Stiffness   ☐ Dull
☐ Other: ──────────

Pain Scale: 1 2 3 4 5 6 7 8 9 10

SYMPTOMS

_____ _____ _____
_____ _____ _____
_____ _____ _____

	PAIN	FATIGUE	ANXIETY	MOOD
AM	/10	/10	/10	/10
PM	/10	/10	/10	/10

TAKEN TODAY

_____ _____ _____
_____ _____ _____
_____ _____ _____

NOTE OF THE DAY

_____
_____
_____

SOMETHING TO MAKE TOMORROW BETTER:

_____
_____
_____

Today's Date : _____

SLEEP _____
_____

BREAKFAST
_____
_____
_____
_____
_____

LUNCH
_____
_____
_____
_____
_____

DINNER
_____
_____
_____
_____
_____

SNACKS
_____
_____
_____

WATER 🥛🥛🥛🥛🥛🥛🥛🥛🥛🥛🥛

TOTAL: _____

ACTIVITIES
_____
_____
_____
_____

How I feel today about my food

○ 🙂   ○ 😐   ○ 🙁

How I feel today about my activities

○ 🙂   ○ 😐   ○ 🙁

Mark the pain zones

Front   Right   Back   Left

Time Started:
Time Ended:
Total Duration:

Type of pain: ☐ Tingling
☐ Shooting ☐ Throbbing
☐ Sharp ☐ Aching ☐ Swelling
☐ Burning ☐ Numbness
☐ Cramping ☐ Stiffness ☐ Dull
☐ Other: ―――――――

Pain Scale: 1 2 3 4 5 6 7 8 9 10

SYMPTOMS

―――――――――――――――――――――――

	PAIN	FATIGUE	ANXIETY	MOOD
AM	/10	/10	/10	/10
PM	/10	/10	/10	/10

TAKEN TODAY

―――――――――――――――――――――――

NOTE OF THE DAY

―――――――――――――――――――――――

SOMETHING TO MAKE TOMORROW BETTER:

―――――――――――――――――――――――

Today's Date: _____

SLEEP _____

BREAKFAST
_____
_____
_____
_____

LUNCH
_____
_____
_____
_____

DINNER
_____
_____
_____
_____

SNACKS
_____
_____
_____

_____
_____
_____

_____
_____
_____

WATER 🥛🥛🥛🥛🥛🥛🥛🥛🥛🥛🥛🥛

TOTAL: _____

ACTIVITIES
_____
_____
_____
_____

How I feel today about my food

○ 🙂   ○ 😐   ○ 🙁

How I feel today about my activities

○ 🙂   ○ 😐   ○ 🙁

Mark the pain zones

Front Right Back Left

Time Started:
Time Ended:
Total Duration:

Type of pain: ☐ Tingling
☐ Shooting   ☐ Throbbing
☐ Sharp ☐ Aching ☐ Swelling
☐ Burning   ☐ Numbness
☐ Cramping ☐ Stiffness ☐ Du
☐ Other: ─────────

Pain Scale: 1 2 3 4 5 6 7 8 9 10

SYMPTOMS

_____ _____ _____
_____ _____ _____
_____ _____ _____

	PAIN	FATIGUE	ANXIETY	MOOD
AM	/10	/10	/10	/10
PM	/10	/10	/10	/10

TAKEN TODAY

_____ _____ _____
_____ _____ _____
_____ _____ _____

NOTE OF THE DAY

_____
_____
_____

SOMETHING TO MAKE TOMORROW BETTER:

_____
_____
_____

Today's Date : _____

SLEEP _____
_____

BREAKFAST   **LUNCH**   **DINNER**
_____   _____   _____
_____   _____   _____
_____   _____   _____
_____   _____   _____
_____   _____   _____

SNACKS
_____   _____   _____
_____   _____   _____
_____   _____   _____

WATER 🍺🍺🍺🍺🍺🍺🍺🍺🍺🍺 🍺🍺
TOTAL: _____

ACTIVITIES
_____
_____
_____
_____

How I feel today about my food

○ 🙂   ○ 😐   ○ 🙁

How I feel today about my activities

○ 🙂   ○ 😐   ○ 🙁

Mark the pain zones

Front Right Back Left

Time Started:
Time Ended:
Total Duration:

Type of pain: ☐ Tingling
☐ Shooting ☐ Throbbing
☐ Sharp ☐ Aching ☐ Swelling
☐ Burning ☐ Numbness
☐ Cramping ☐ Stiffness ☐ Dull
☐ Other: ─────────

Pain Scale: 1 2 3 4 5 6 7 8 9 10

SYMPTOMS

	PAIN	FATIGUE	ANXIETY	MOOD
AM	/10	/10	/10	/10
PM	/10	/10	/10	/10

TAKEN TODAY

NOTE OF THE DAY

SOMETHING TO MAKE TOMORROW BETTER:

Stronger than you Think

Today's Date: _____

SLEEP _____

BREAKFAST

LUNCH

DINNER

SNACKS

WATER 🥛🥛🥛🥛🥛🥛🥛🥛🥛🥛🥛🥛🥛

TOTAL: _____

ACTIVITIES

How I feel today about my food

○ 🙂   ○ 😐   ○ 🙁

How I feel today about my activities

○ 🙂   ○ 😐   ○ 🙁

Mark the pain zones

Front   Right   Back   Left

Time Started:
Time Ended:
Total Duration:

Type of pain: ☐ Tingling
☐ Shooting ☐ Throbbing
☐ Sharp ☐ Aching ☐ Swelling
☐ Burning ☐ Numbness
☐ Cramping ☐ Stiffness ☐ Dull
☐ Other: _____

Pain Scale: |—1—|—2—|—3—|—4—|—5—|—6—|—7—|—8—|—9—|—10—|

SYMPTOMS

_____ _____ _____
_____ _____ _____
_____ _____ _____

	PAIN	FATIGUE	ANXIETY	MOOD
AM	/10	/10	/10	/10
PM	/10	/10	/10	/10

TAKEN TODAY

_____ _____ _____
_____ _____ _____
_____ _____ _____

NOTE OF THE DAY

_____
_____
_____

SOMETHING TO MAKE TOMORROW BETTER:

_____
_____
_____

Today's Date: _____

SLEEP _____

BREAKFAST
_____
_____
_____
_____
_____

LUNCH
_____
_____
_____
_____
_____

DINNER
_____
_____
_____
_____
_____

SNACKS
_____
_____
_____
_____

WATER 🥛🥛🥛🥛🥛🥛🥛🥛🥛🥛🥛🥛

TOTAL: _____

ACTIVITIES
_____
_____
_____
_____

How I feel today about my food

○ 🙂   ○ 😐   ○ 🙁

How I feel today about my activities

○ 🙂   ○ 😐   ○ 🙁

Mark the pain zones

Front Right Back Left

Time Started:
Time Ended:
Total Duration:

Type of pain: ☐ Tingling
☐ Shooting ☐ Throbbing
☐ Sharp ☐ Aching ☐ Swelling
☐ Burning ☐ Numbness
☐ Cramping ☐ Stiffness ☐ Dull
☐ Other: ─────────

Pain Scale: 1 2 3 4 5 6 7 8 9 10

SYMPTOMS

_____   _____   _____
_____   _____   _____
_____   _____   _____

	PAIN	FATIGUE	ANXIETY	MOOD
AM	/10	/10	/10	/10
PM	/10	/10	/10	/10

TAKEN TODAY

_____   _____   _____
_____   _____   _____
_____   _____   _____

NOTE OF THE DAY

_____
_____
_____

SOMETHING TO MAKE TOMORROW BETTER:

_____
_____
_____

Today's Date : _____

SLEEP _____
_____

BREAKFAST
_____
_____
_____
_____
_____

LUNCH
_____
_____
_____
_____
_____

DINNER
_____
_____
_____
_____
_____

SNACKS
_____
_____
_____

WATER 🥤🥤🥤🥤🥤🥤🥤🥤🥤🥤🥤🥤
TOTAL: _____

ACTIVITIES
_____
_____
_____

How I feel today about my food

○    ○   ○

How I feel today about my activities

○   ○   ○

Mark the pain zones

Front Right Back Left

Time Started:
Time Ended:
Total Duration:

Type of pain: ☐ Tingling
☐ Shooting ☐ Throbbing
☐ Sharp ☐ Aching ☐ Swelling
☐ Burning ☐ Numbness
☐ Cramping ☐ Stiffness ☐ Dull
☐ Other: ―――――――――

Pain Scale: 1 2 3 4 5 6 7 8 9 10

SYMPTOMS

――――――――― ――――――――― ―――――――――
――――――――― ――――――――― ―――――――――
――――――――― ――――――――― ―――――――――

	PAIN	FATIGUE	ANXIETY	MOOD
AM	/10	/10	/10	/10
PM	/10	/10	/10	/10

TAKEN TODAY

――――――――― ――――――――― ―――――――――
――――――――― ――――――――― ―――――――――
――――――――― ――――――――― ―――――――――

NOTE OF THE DAY

―――――――――――――――――――――――――――――
―――――――――――――――――――――――――――――
―――――――――――――――――――――――――――――

SOMETHING TO MAKE TOMORROW BETTER:

―――――――――――――――――――――――――――――
―――――――――――――――――――――――――――――
―――――――――――――――――――――――――――――

Today's Date: _____

SLEEP _____
_____

BREAKFAST
_____
_____
_____
_____

LUNCH
_____
_____
_____
_____

DINNER
_____
_____
_____
_____

SNACKS
_____ _____ _____
_____ _____ _____

WATER 🥛 🥛 🥛 🥛 🥛 🥛 🥛 🥛 🥛 🥛 🥛 🥛

TOTAL: _____

ACTIVITIES
_____
_____
_____

How I feel today about my food

○ 🙂   ○ 😐   ○ 🙁

How I feel today about my activities

○ 🙂   ○ 😐   ○ 🙁

Mark the pain zones

Front Right Back Left

Time Started:
Time Ended:
Total Duration:

Type of pain: ☐ Tingling
☐ Shooting ☐ Throbbing
☐ Sharp ☐ Aching ☐ Swelling
☐ Burning ☐ Numbness
☐ Cramping ☐ Stiffness ☐ Dull
☐ Other: ──────

Pain Scale: 1 2 3 4 5 6 7 8 9 10

SYMPTOMS

	PAIN	FATIGUE	ANXIETY	MOOD
AM	/10	/10	/10	/10
PM	/10	/10	/10	/10

TAKEN TODAY

NOTE OF THE DAY

SOMETHING TO MAKE TOMORROW BETTER:

Today's Date: _____

SLEEP _____
_____

BREAKFAST   LUNCH   DINNER
_____   _____   _____
_____   _____   _____
_____   _____   _____
_____   _____   _____

SNACKS
_____   _____   _____
_____   _____   _____
_____   _____   _____

WATER 🥛🥛🥛🥛🥛🥛🥛🥛🥛🥛🥛🥛
TOTAL: _____

ACTIVITIES
_____
_____
_____
_____

How I feel today about my food

○ 🙂   ○ 😐   ○ 🙁

How I feel today about my activities

○ 🙂   ○ 😐   ○ 🙁

Mark the pain zones

Front Right Back Left

Time Started:
Time Ended:
Total Duration:

Type of pain: ☐ Tingling
☐ Shooting ☐ Throbbing
☐ Sharp ☐ Aching ☐ Swelling
☐ Burning ☐ Numbness
☐ Cramping ☐ Stiffness ☐ Dull
☐ Other: ─────────

Pain Scale: 1 2 3 4 5 6 7 8 9 10

SYMPTOMS

_____ _____ _____
_____ _____ _____
_____ _____ _____

	PAIN	FATIGUE	ANXIETY	MOOD
AM	/10	/10	/10	/10
PM	/10	/10	/10	/10

TAKEN TODAY

_____ _____ _____
_____ _____ _____
_____ _____ _____

NOTE OF THE DAY

_____
_____
_____

SOMETHING TO MAKE TOMORROW BETTER:

_____
_____
_____

Today's Date : _____

SLEEP _____
_____

BREAKFAST   LUNCH   DINNER
_____   _____   _____
_____   _____   _____
_____   _____   _____
_____   _____   _____
_____   _____   _____

SNACKS
_____   _____   _____
_____   _____   _____
_____   _____   _____

WATER 🥛🥛🥛🥛🥛🥛🥛🥛🥛🥛🥛🥛
                                    TOTAL: _____

ACTIVITIES
_____
_____
_____
_____

How I feel today about my food

　　o 🙂　　　o 😐　　　o 🙁

How I feel today about my activities

　　o 🙂　　　o 😐　　　o 🙁

Mark the pain zones

Front   Right   Back   Left

Time Started:
Time Ended:
Total Duration:

Type of pain: ☐ Tingling
☐ Shooting ☐ Throbbing
☐ Sharp ☐ Aching ☐ Swelling
☐ Burning ☐ Numbness
☐ Cramping ☐ Stiffness ☐ Dull
☐ Other: ─────────

Pain Scale: 1 2 3 4 5 6 7 8 9 10

SYMPTOMS

_____ _____ _____
_____ _____ _____
_____ _____ _____

	PAIN	FATIGUE	ANXIETY	MOOD
AM	/10	/10	/10	/10
PM	/10	/10	/10	/10

TAKEN TODAY

_____ _____ _____
_____ _____ _____
_____ _____ _____

NOTE OF THE DAY

_____
_____
_____

SOMETHING TO MAKE TOMORROW BETTER:

_____
_____
_____

Today's Date: _____

SLEEP
_____
_____

BREAKFAST
_____
_____
_____
_____
_____

LUNCH
_____
_____
_____
_____
_____

DINNER
_____
_____
_____
_____
_____

SNACKS
_____
_____
_____

WATER 🥛🥛🥛🥛🥛🥛🥛🥛🥛🥛🥛🥛
TOTAL: _____

ACTIVITIES
_____
_____
_____
_____

How I feel today about my food
○ 🙂   ○ 😐   ○ ☹️

How I feel today about my activities
○ 🙂   ○ 😐   ○ ☹️

Mark the pain zones

Front Right Back Left

Time Started:
Time Ended:
Total Duration:

Type of pain: ☐ Tingling
☐ Shooting ☐ Throbbing
☐ Sharp ☐ Aching ☐ Swelling
☐ Burning ☐ Numbness
☐ Cramping ☐ Stiffness ☐ Dull
☐ Other: ──────────

Pain Scale: 1 2 3 4 5 6 7 8 9 10

SYMPTOMS

_____ _____ _____
_____ _____ _____
_____ _____

	PAIN	FATIGUE	ANXIETY	MOOD
AM	/10	/10	/10	/10
PM	/10	/10	/10	/10

TAKEN TODAY

_____ _____ _____
_____ _____ _____
_____ _____

NOTE OF THE DAY

_____
_____
_____

SOMETHING TO MAKE TOMORROW BETTER:

_____
_____
_____

Today's Date : _____

SLEEP _____

BREAKFAST
_____
_____
_____
_____
_____

LUNCH
_____
_____
_____
_____
_____

DINNER
_____
_____
_____
_____
_____

SNACKS
_____
_____
_____

WATER 🥛🥛🥛🥛🥛🥛🥛🥛🥛🥛🥛🥛

TOTAL: _____

ACTIVITIES
_____
_____
_____
_____

How I feel today about my food

○ 🙂   ○ 😐   ○ ☹️

How I feel today about my activities

○ 🙂   ○ 😐   ○ ☹️

Mark the pain zones

Front Right Back Left

Time Started:
Time Ended:
Total Duration:

Type of pain: ☐ Tingling
☐ Shooting ☐ Throbbing
☐ Sharp ☐ Aching ☐ Swelling
☐ Burning ☐ Numbness
☐ Cramping ☐ Stiffness ☐ Dull
☐ Other: ─────────

Pain Scale: 1 2 3 4 5 6 7 8 9 10

SYMPTOMS

	PAIN	FATIGUE	ANXIETY	MOOD
AM	/10	/10	/10	/10
PM	/10	/10	/10	/10

TAKEN TODAY

NOTE OF THE DAY

SOMETHING TO MAKE TOMORROW BETTER:

The strongest people are those who win battles you know nothing about

Today's Date : _____

SLEEP _____

BREAKFAST
_____
_____
_____
_____

LUNCH
_____
_____
_____
_____

DINNER
_____
_____
_____
_____

SNACKS
_____
_____
_____

WATER 🥛🥛🥛🥛🥛🥛🥛🥛🥛🥛🥛🥛

TOTAL: _____

ACTIVITIES
_____
_____
_____

How I feel today about my food

○ 🙂   ○ 😐   ○ 🙁

How I feel today about my activities

○ 🙂   ○ 😐   ○ 🙁

Mark the pain zones

Front Right Back Left

Time Started:
Time Ended:
Total Duration:

Type of pain: ☐ Tingling
☐ Shooting ☐ Throbbing
☐ Sharp ☐ Aching ☐ Swelling
☐ Burning ☐ Numbness
☐ Cramping ☐ Stiffness ☐ Du
☐ Other: ─────────

Pain Scale: 1 2 3 4 5 6 7 8 9 10

SYMPTOMS

	PAIN	FATIGUE	ANXIETY	MOOD
AM	/10	/10	/10	/10
PM	/10	/10	/10	/10

TAKEN TODAY

NOTE OF THE DAY

SOMETHING TO MAKE TOMORROW BETTER:

Today's Date : _____

SLEEP
_____
_____

BREAKFAST
_____
_____
_____
_____
_____

LUNCH
_____
_____
_____
_____
_____

DINNER
_____
_____
_____
_____
_____

SNACKS
_____
_____
_____

WATER 🥤🥤🥤🥤🥤🥤🥤🥤🥤🥤🥤🥤

TOTAL: _____

ACTIVITIES
_____
_____
_____

How I feel today about my food

○ 🙂   ○ 😐   ○ ☹️

How I feel today about my activities

○ 🙂   ○ 😐   ○ ☹️

Mark the pain zones

Front Right Back Left

Time Started:
Time Ended:
Total Duration:

Type of pain: ☐ Tingling
☐ Shooting ☐ Throbbing
☐ Sharp ☐ Aching ☐ Swelling
☐ Burning ☐ Numbness
☐ Cramping ☐ Stiffness ☐ Dull
☐ Other: ─────────

Pain Scale: 1 2 3 4 5 6 7 8 9 10

SYMPTOMS

_____ _____ _____
_____ _____ _____
_____ _____ _____

	PAIN	FATIGUE	ANXIETY	MOOD
AM	/10	/10	/10	/10
PM	/10	/10	/10	/10

TAKEN TODAY

_____ _____ _____
_____ _____ _____
_____ _____ _____

NOTE OF THE DAY

_____
_____
_____

SOMETHING TO MAKE TOMORROW BETTER:

_____
_____
_____

Today's Date : _____

SLEEP _____

BREAKFAST   **LUNCH**   **DINNER**

SNACKS

WATER 🥛🥛🥛🥛🥛🥛🥛🥛🥛🥛🥛   TOTAL: _____

ACTIVITIES

How I feel today about my food

○ 🙂   ○ 😐   ○ ☹️

How I feel today about my activities

○ 🙂   ○ 😐   ○ ☹️

Mark the pain zones

Time Started:
Time Ended:
Total Duration:

Type of pain: ☐ Tingling
☐ Shooting ☐ Throbbing
☐ Sharp ☐ Aching ☐ Swelling
☐ Burning ☐ Numbness
☐ Cramping ☐ Stiffness ☐ Dull
☐ Other: ─────────

Front   Right   Back   Left

Pain Scale: 1 2 3 4 5 6 7 8 9 10

SYMPTOMS

_____ _____ _____
_____ _____ _____
_____

	PAIN	FATIGUE	ANXIETY	MOOD
AM	/10	/10	/10	/10
PM	/10	/10	/10	/10

TAKEN TODAY

_____ _____ _____
_____ _____ _____
_____

NOTE OF THE DAY

_____
_____
_____

SOMETHING TO MAKE TOMORROW BETTER:

_____
_____
_____

Today's Date : _____

SLEEP
_____
_____

BREAKFAST
_____
_____
_____
_____
_____

LUNCH
_____
_____
_____
_____
_____

DINNER
_____
_____
_____
_____
_____

SNACKS
_____
_____
_____

_____
_____
_____

_____
_____
_____

WATER 🥛🥛🥛🥛🥛🥛🥛🥛🥛🥛🥛🥛

TOTAL: _____

ACTIVITIES
_____
_____
_____

How I feel today about my food

○ 🙂   ○ 😐   ○ ☹️

How I feel today about my activities

○ 🙂   ○ 😐   ○ ☹️

Mark the pain zones

Front Right Back Left

Time Started:
Time Ended:
Total Duration:

Type of pain: ☐ Tingling
☐ Shooting ☐ Throbbing
☐ Sharp ☐ Aching ☐ Swelling
☐ Burning ☐ Numbness
☐ Cramping ☐ Stiffness ☐ Du
☐ Other: ─────────────

Pain Scale: 1 2 3 4 5 6 7 8 9 10

SYMPTOMS

_____ _____ _____
_____ _____ _____
_____ _____ _____

	PAIN	FATIGUE	ANXIETY	MOOD
AM	/10	/10	/10	/10
PM	/10	/10	/10	/10

TAKEN TODAY

_____ _____ _____
_____ _____ _____
_____ _____ _____

NOTE OF THE DAY

_____
_____
_____

SOMETHING TO MAKE TOMORROW BETTER:

_____
_____
_____

Today's Date : _____

SLEEP _____
_____

BREAKFAST
_____
_____
_____
_____
_____

LUNCH
_____
_____
_____
_____
_____

DINNER
_____
_____
_____
_____
_____

SNACKS
_____
_____
_____

_____
_____
_____

WATER 🥛🥛🥛🥛🥛🥛🥛🥛🥛🥛🥛🥛

TOTAL: _____

ACTIVITIES
_____
_____
_____
_____

How I feel today about my food

○ 🙂   ○ 😐   ○ ☹️

How I feel today about my activities

○ 🙂   ○ 😐   ○ ☹️

Mark the pain zones

Front Right Back Left

Time Started:
Time Ended:
Total Duration:

Type of pain: ☐ Tingling
☐ Shooting ☐ Throbbing
☐ Sharp ☐ Aching ☐ Swelling
☐ Burning ☐ Numbness
☐ Cramping ☐ Stiffness ☐ Dull
☐ Other: ─────────

Pain Scale: 1 2 3 4 5 6 7 8 9 10

SYMPTOMS

	PAIN	FATIGUE	ANXIETY	MOOD
AM	/10	/10	/10	/10
PM	/10	/10	/10	/10

TAKEN TODAY

NOTE OF THE DAY

SOMETHING TO MAKE TOMORROW BETTER:

Today's Date : _____

SLEEP _____

BREAKFAST	LUNCH	DINNER
_____	_____	_____
_____	_____	_____
_____	_____	_____
_____	_____	_____

SNACKS
_____   _____   _____
_____   _____   _____
_____   _____   _____

WATER 🥛🥛🥛🥛🥛🥛🥛🥛🥛🥛🥛🥛

TOTAL: _____

ACTIVITIES
_____
_____
_____

How I feel today about my food

○ 🙂   ○ 😐   ○ 🙁

How I feel today about my activities

○ 🙂   ○ 😐   ○ 🙁

Mark the pain zones

Front   Right   Back   Left

Time Started:
Time Ended:
Total Duration:

Type of pain: ☐ Tingling
☐ Shooting   ☐ Throbbing
☐ Sharp   ☐ Aching   ☐ Swelling
☐ Burning   ☐ Numbness
☐ Cramping   ☐ Stiffness   ☐ Dull
☐ Other: _____

Pain Scale: 1 2 3 4 5 6 7 8 9 10

SYMPTOMS

_____   _____   _____
_____   _____   _____
_____

	PAIN	FATIGUE	ANXIETY	MOOD
AM	/10	/10	/10	/10
PM	/10	/10	/10	/10

TAKEN TODAY

_____   _____   _____
_____   _____   _____

NOTE OF THE DAY

_____
_____
_____

SOMETHING TO MAKE TOMORROW BETTER:

_____
_____
_____

Today's Date : _____

```
SLEEP  _____
       _____
```

BREAKFAST   LUNCH   DINNER
_____   _____   _____
_____   _____   _____
_____   _____   _____
_____   _____   _____

SNACKS
_____   _____   _____
_____   _____   _____
_____   _____   _____

WATER 🥛🥛🥛🥛🥛🥛🥛🥛🥛🥛🥛🥛
                              TOTAL: _____

ACTIVITIES
_____
_____
_____
_____

How I feel today about my food

  ○ 🙂   ○ 😐   ○ 🙁

How I feel today about my activities

  ○ 🙂   ○ 😐   ○ 🙁

Mark the pain zones

Front   Right   Back   Left

Time Started:
Time Ended:
Total Duration:

Type of pain: ☐ Tingling
☐ Shooting ☐ Throbbing
☐ Sharp ☐ Aching ☐ Swelling
☐ Burning ☐ Numbness
☐ Cramping ☐ Stiffness ☐ Du
☐ Other: ─────────

Pain Scale: 1 2 3 4 5 6 7 8 9 10

SYMPTOMS

	PAIN	FATIGUE	ANXIETY	MOOD
AM	/10	/10	/10	/10
PM	/10	/10	/10	/10

TAKEN TODAY

NOTE OF THE DAY

SOMETHING TO MAKE TOMORROW BETTER:

Today's Date: _____

SLEEP _____
_____

BREAKFAST
_____
_____
_____
_____
_____

LUNCH
_____
_____
_____
_____
_____

DINNER
_____
_____
_____
_____
_____

SNACKS
_____
_____
_____

WATER 🥛 🥛 🥛 🥛 🥛 🥛 🥛 🥛 🥛 🥛 🥛 🥛

TOTAL: _____

ACTIVITIES
_____
_____
_____

How I feel today about my food

○ 🙂   ○ 😐   ○ 🙁

How I feel today about my activities

○ 🙂   ○ 😐   ○ 🙁

Mark the pain zones

Front   Right   Back   Left

Time Started:
Time Ended:
Total Duration:

Type of pain: ☐ Tingling
☐ Shooting ☐ Throbbing
☐ Sharp ☐ Aching ☐ Swelling
☐ Burning ☐ Numbness
☐ Cramping ☐ Stiffness ☐ Dull
☐ Other: ―――――――

Pain Scale: 1 2 3 4 5 6 7 8 9 10

SYMPTOMS

_____
_____
_____

	PAIN	FATIGUE	ANXIETY	MOOD
AM	/10	/10	/10	/10
PM	/10	/10	/10	/10

TAKEN TODAY

_____
_____
_____

NOTE OF THE DAY

_____
_____
_____

SOMETHING TO MAKE TOMORROW BETTER:

_____
_____
_____

If I can survive the war that I battle with myself I can survive Anything

Today's Date : _____

SLEEP _____
_____

BREAKFAST   LUNCH   DINNER
_____   _____   _____
_____   _____   _____
_____   _____   _____
_____   _____   _____
_____   _____   _____

SNACKS
_____   _____   _____
_____   _____   _____
_____   _____   _____

WATER 🥛🥛🥛🥛🥛🥛🥛🥛🥛🥛🥛🥛🥛
TOTAL: _____

ACTIVITIES
_____
_____
_____
_____

How I feel today about my food

  o 🙂   o 😐   o 🙁

How I feel today about my activities

  o 🙂   o 😐   o 🙁

Mark the pain zones

Front Right Back Left

Time Started:
Time Ended:
Total Duration:

Type of pain: ☐ Tingling
☐ Shooting ☐ Throbbing
☐ Sharp ☐ Aching ☐ Swelling
☐ Burning ☐ Numbness
☐ Cramping ☐ Stiffness ☐ Du
☐ Other: ─────────

Pain Scale: 1 2 3 4 5 6 7 8 9 10

SYMPTOMS

_____ _____ _____
_____ _____ _____
_____ _____ _____

	PAIN	FATIGUE	ANXIETY	MOOD
AM	/10	/10	/10	/10
PM	/10	/10	/10	/10

TAKEN TODAY

_____ _____ _____
_____ _____ _____
_____ _____ _____

NOTE OF THE DAY

_____
_____
_____

SOMETHING TO MAKE TOMORROW BETTER:

_____
_____
_____

Today's Date : _____

SLEEP _____
_____

BREAKFAST   **LUNCH**   **DINNER**
_____   _____   _____
_____   _____   _____
_____   _____   _____
_____   _____   _____

SNACKS
_____   _____   _____
_____   _____   _____

WATER 🥛🥛🥛🥛🥛🥛🥛🥛🥛🥛🥛
TOTAL: _____

ACTIVITIES
_____
_____
_____

How I feel today about my food

○ 🙂   ○ 😐   ○ 🙁

How I feel today about my activities

○ 🙂   ○ 😐   ○ 🙁

Mark the pain zones

Front   Right   Back   Left

Pain Scale: 1 2 3 4 5 6 7 8 9 10

Time Started:
Time Ended:
Total Duration:

Type of pain: ☐ Tingling
☐ Shooting   ☐ Throbbing
☐ Sharp ☐ Aching ☐ Swelling
☐ Burning   ☐ Numbness
☐ Cramping ☐ Stiffness ☐ Dull
☐ Other: ─────────────

SYMPTOMS

	PAIN	FATIGUE	ANXIETY	MOOD
AM	/10	/10	/10	/10
PM	/10	/10	/10	/10

TAKEN TODAY

NOTE OF THE DAY

SOMETHING TO MAKE TOMORROW BETTER:

Today's Date: _____

SLEEP _____

BREAKFAST
_____
_____
_____
_____

LUNCH
_____
_____
_____
_____

DINNER
_____
_____
_____
_____

SNACKS
_____
_____

_____
_____

_____
_____

WATER 🥛🥛🥛🥛🥛🥛🥛🥛🥛🥛   **TOTAL:** _____

ACTIVITIES
_____
_____
_____

How I feel today about my food
  ○ 🙂   ○ 😐   ○ 🙁

How I feel today about my activities
  ○ 🙂   ○ 😐   ○ 🙁

Mark the pain zones

Front   Right   Back   Left

Time Started:
Time Ended:
Total Duration:

Type of pain: ☐ Tingling
☐ Shooting ☐ Throbbing
☐ Sharp ☐ Aching ☐ Swelling
☐ Burning   ☐ Numbness
☐ Cramping ☐ Stiffness ☐ Dull
☐ Other: ─────────

Pain Scale: 1 2 3 4 5 6 7 8 9 10

SYMPTOMS

	PAIN	FATIGUE	ANXIETY	MOOD
AM	/10	/10	/10	/10
PM	/10	/10	/10	/10

TAKEN TODAY

NOTE OF THE DAY

SOMETHING TO MAKE TOMORROW BETTER:

Today's Date : _____

SLEEP _____
_____

BREAKFAST
_____
_____
_____
_____
_____

LUNCH
_____
_____
_____
_____
_____

DINNER
_____
_____
_____
_____
_____

SNACKS
_____
_____
_____

_____
_____
_____

_____
_____
_____

WATER 🥛🥛🥛🥛🥛🥛🥛🥛🥛🥛🥛🥛

TOTAL: _____

ACTIVITIES
_____
_____
_____
_____

How I feel today about my food

o 🙂   o 😐   o 🙁

How I feel today about my activities

o 🙂   o 😐   o 🙁

Mark the pain zones

Front Right Back Left

Time Started:
Time Ended:
Total Duration:

Type of pain: ☐ Tingling
☐ Shooting ☐ Throbbing
☐ Sharp ☐ Aching ☐ Swelling
☐ Burning ☐ Numbness
☐ Cramping ☐ Stiffness ☐ Du
☐ Other: ─────────

Pain Scale: 1 2 3 4 5 6 7 8 9 10

SYMPTOMS

_____ _____ _____
_____ _____ _____
_____ _____ _____

	PAIN	FATIGUE	ANXIETY	MOOD
AM	/10	/10	/10	/10
PM	/10	/10	/10	/10

TAKEN TODAY

_____ _____ _____
_____ _____ _____
_____ _____ _____

NOTE OF THE DAY

_____
_____
_____

SOMETHING TO MAKE TOMORROW BETTER:

_____
_____
_____

Today's Date : _____

SLEEP _____
_____

BREAKFAST
_____
_____
_____
_____
_____

LUNCH
_____
_____
_____
_____
_____

DINNER
_____
_____
_____
_____
_____

SNACKS
_____
_____
_____

WATER 🍺🍺🍺🍺🍺🍺🍺🍺🍺🍺🍺🍺

TOTAL: _____

ACTIVITIES
_____
_____
_____

How I feel today about my food

○ 🙂   ○ 😐   ○ ☹️

How I feel today about my activities

○ 🙂   ○ 😐   ○ ☹️

Mark the pain zones

Front   Right   Back   Left

Time Started:
Time Ended:
Total Duration:

Type of pain: ☐ Tingling
☐ Shooting   ☐ Throbbing
☐ Sharp ☐ Aching ☐ Swelling
☐ Burning   ☐ Numbness
☐ Cramping ☐ Stiffness ☐ Dull
☐ Other: ─────────────

Pain Scale: 1 2 3 4 5 6 7 8 9 10

SYMPTOMS

	PAIN	FATIGUE	ANXIETY	MOOD
AM	/10	/10	/10	/10
PM	/10	/10	/10	/10

TAKEN TODAY

NOTE OF THE DAY

SOMETHING TO MAKE TOMORROW BETTER:

Today's Date : _____

SLEEP _____
_____

BREAKFAST
_____
_____
_____
_____
_____

LUNCH
_____
_____
_____
_____
_____

DINNER
_____
_____
_____
_____
_____

SNACKS
_____ _____ _____
_____ _____ _____

WATER 🍺🍺🍺🍺🍺🍺🍺🍺🍺🍺

TOTAL: _____

ACTIVITIES
_____
_____
_____

How I feel today about my food

○ 🙂   ○ 😐   ○ 🙁

How I feel today about my activities

○ 🙂   ○ 😐   ○ 🙁

Mark the pain zones

Front Right Back Left

Time Started:
Time Ended:
Total Duration:

Type of pain: ☐ Tingling
☐ Shooting ☐ Throbbing
☐ Sharp ☐ Aching ☐ Swelling
☐ Burning ☐ Numbness
☐ Cramping ☐ Stiffness ☐ Dull
☐ Other: _____

Pain Scale: 1 2 3 4 5 6 7 8 9 10

SYMPTOMS

_____ _____ _____
_____ _____ _____
_____ _____ _____

	PAIN	FATIGUE	ANXIETY	MOOD
AM	/10	/10	/10	/10
PM	/10	/10	/10	/10

TAKEN TODAY

_____ _____ _____
_____ _____ _____
_____ _____ _____

NOTE OF THE DAY

_____
_____
_____

SOMETHING TO MAKE TOMORROW BETTER:

_____
_____
_____

Today's Date: _____

SLEEP _____

BREAKFAST
_____
_____
_____
_____
_____

LUNCH
_____
_____
_____
_____
_____

DINNER
_____
_____
_____
_____
_____

SNACKS
_____
_____
_____

WATER 🥛🥛🥛🥛🥛🥛🥛🥛🥛🥛🥛🥛

TOTAL: ____

ACTIVITIES
_____
_____
_____
_____

How I feel today about my food

○ 🙂   ○ 😐   ○ 🙁

How I feel today about my activities

○ 🙂   ○ 😐   ○ 🙁

Mark the pain zones

Front Right Back Left

Time Started:
Time Ended:
Total Duration:

Type of pain: ☐ Tingling
☐ Shooting ☐ Throbbing
☐ Sharp ☐ Aching ☐ Swelling
☐ Burning ☐ Numbness
☐ Cramping ☐ Stiffness ☐ Du
☐ Other: ─────────

Pain Scale: 1 2 3 4 5 6 7 8 9 10

SYMPTOMS

	PAIN	FATIGUE	ANXIETY	MOOD
AM	/10	/10	/10	/10
PM	/10	/10	/10	/10

TAKEN TODAY

NOTE OF THE DAY

SOMETHING TO MAKE TOMORROW BETTER:

Today's Date: _____

SLEEP _____

BREAKFAST	LUNCH	DINNER
_____	_____	_____
_____	_____	_____
_____	_____	_____
_____	_____	_____
_____	_____	_____

SNACKS
_____
_____
_____

WATER 🥛🥛🥛🥛🥛🥛🥛🥛🥛🥛🥛🥛   TOTAL: _____

ACTIVITIES
_____
_____
_____

How I feel today about my food

○ 🙂   ○ 😐   ○ 🙁

How I feel today about my activities

○ 🙂   ○ 😐   ○ 🙁

Mark the pain zones

Front   Right   Back   Left

Time Started:
Time Ended:
Total Duration:

Type of pain:
☐ Tingling ☐ Shooting ☐ Throbbing
☐ Sharp ☐ Aching ☐ Swelling
☐ Burning ☐ Numbness
☐ Cramping ☐ Stiffness ☐ Dull
☐ Other: _____

Pain Scale: 1 2 3 4 5 6 7 8 9 10

SYMPTOMS

	PAIN	FATIGUE	ANXIETY	MOOD
AM	/10	/10	/10	/10
PM	/10	/10	/10	/10

TAKEN TODAY

NOTE OF THE DAY

SOMETHING TO MAKE TOMORROW BETTER:

Fighting Every Single Day

Today's Date: _____

SLEEP _____
_____

BREAKFAST
_____
_____
_____
_____
_____

LUNCH
_____
_____
_____
_____
_____

DINNER
_____
_____
_____
_____
_____

SNACKS
_____
_____
_____

_____
_____
_____

_____
_____
_____

WATER 🥤🥤🥤🥤🥤🥤🥤🥤🥤🥤🥤🥤

TOTAL: _____

ACTIVITIES
_____
_____
_____
_____

How I feel today about my food

○ 🙂   ○ 😐   ○ 🙁

How I feel today about my activities

○ 🙂   ○ 😐   ○ 🙁

Mark the pain zones

Front Right Back Left

Time Started:
Time Ended:
Total Duration:

Type of pain: ☐ Tingling
☐ Shooting ☐ Throbbing
☐ Sharp ☐ Aching ☐ Swelling
☐ Burning ☐ Numbness
☐ Cramping ☐ Stiffness ☐ Du
☐ Other: ─────────────

Pain Scale: 1 2 3 4 5 6 7 8 9 10

SYMPTOMS

	PAIN	FATIGUE	ANXIETY	MOOD
AM	/10	/10	/10	/10
PM	/10	/10	/10	/10

TAKEN TODAY

NOTE OF THE DAY

SOMETHING TO MAKE TOMORROW BETTER:

Today's Date : _____

SLEEP _____
      _____

BREAKFAST   LUNCH   DINNER
_____   _____   _____
_____   _____   _____
_____   _____   _____
_____   _____   _____
_____   _____   _____

SNACKS
_____   _____   _____
_____   _____   _____
_____   _____   _____

WATER 🍺 🍺 🍺 🍺 🍺 🍺 🍺 🍺 🍺 🍺 🍺
                                        TOTAL: _____

ACTIVITIES
_____
_____
_____
_____

How I feel today about my food

   o   🙂   o   😐   o   🙁

How I feel today about my activities

   o   🙂   o   😐   o   🙁

Mark the pain zones

Front Right Back Left

Time Started:
Time Ended:
Total Duration:

Type of pain: ☐ Tingling
☐ Shooting ☐ Throbbing
☐ Sharp ☐ Aching ☐ Swelling
☐ Burning ☐ Numbness
☐ Cramping ☐ Stiffness ☐ Dull
☐ Other: ─────────

Pain Scale: 1 2 3 4 5 6 7 8 9 10

SYMPTOMS

_____ _____ _____
_____ _____ _____
_____ _____ _____

	PAIN	FATIGUE	ANXIETY	MOOD
AM	/10	/10	/10	/10
PM	/10	/10	/10	/10

TAKEN TODAY

_____ _____ _____
_____ _____ _____

NOTE OF THE DAY

_____
_____
_____

SOMETHING TO MAKE TOMORROW BETTER:

_____
_____
_____

Today's Date : _____

SLEEP _____
_____

BREAKFAST
_____
_____
_____
_____

LUNCH
_____
_____
_____
_____

DINNER
_____
_____
_____
_____

SNACKS
_____   _____   _____
_____   _____   _____

WATER 🥛 🥛 🥛 🥛 🥛 🥛 🥛 🥛 🥛 🥛 🥛 🥛

TOTAL: _____

ACTIVITIES
_____
_____
_____
_____

How I feel today about my food

○ 🙂   ○ 😐   ○ 🙁

How I feel today about my activities

○ 🙂   ○ 😐   ○ 🙁

Mark the pain zones

Front Right Back Left

Time Started:
Time Ended:
Total Duration:

Type of pain: ☐ Tingling
☐ Shooting ☐ Throbbing
☐ Sharp ☐ Aching ☐ Swelling
☐ Burning ☐ Numbness
☐ Cramping ☐ Stiffness ☐ Dull
☐ Other: ——————————

Pain Scale: 1 2 3 4 5 6 7 8 9 10

SYMPTOMS

_____ _____ _____
_____ _____ _____
_____ _____

	PAIN	FATIGUE	ANXIETY	MOOD
AM	/10	/10	/10	/10
PM	/10	/10	/10	/10

TAKEN TODAY

NOTE OF THE DAY

SOMETHING TO MAKE TOMORROW BETTER:

Today's Date : _____

SLEEP _____
_____

BREAKFAST
_____
_____
_____
_____
_____

LUNCH
_____
_____
_____
_____
_____

DINNER
_____
_____
_____
_____
_____

SNACKS
_____
_____
_____

_____
_____
_____

_____
_____
_____

WATER 🥤🥤🥤🥤🥤🥤🥤🥤🥤🥤🥤🥤
TOTAL: _____

ACTIVITIES
_____
_____
_____
_____

How I feel today about my food

○ 🙂   ○ 😐   ○ 🙁

How I feel today about my activities

○ 🙂   ○ 😐   ○ 🙁

Mark the pain zones

Front Right Back Left

Time Started:
Time Ended:
Total Duration:

Type of pain: ☐ Tingling
☐ Shooting ☐ Throbbing
☐ Sharp ☐ Aching ☐ Swelling
☐ Burning ☐ Numbness
☐ Cramping ☐ Stiffness ☐ Du
☐ Other: ――――――

Pain Scale: 1 2 3 4 5 6 7 8 9 10

SYMPTOMS

_____   _____   _____
_____   _____   _____
_____   _____   _____

	PAIN	FATIGUE	ANXIETY	MOOD
AM	/10	/10	/10	/10
PM	/10	/10	/10	/10

TAKEN TODAY

_____   _____   _____
_____   _____   _____
_____   _____   _____

NOTE OF THE DAY

_____
_____
_____

SOMETHING TO MAKE TOMORROW BETTER:

_____
_____
_____

Today's Date: _____

SLEEP _____
_____

BREAKFAST   **LUNCH**   **DINNER**
_____   _____   _____
_____   _____   _____
_____   _____   _____
_____   _____   _____
_____   _____   _____

SNACKS
_____   _____   _____
_____   _____   _____

WATER 🥛 🥛 🥛 🥛 🥛 🥛 🥛 🥛 🥛 🥛 🥛
TOTAL: _____

ACTIVITIES
_____
_____
_____

How I feel today about my food

○ 🙂   ○ 😐   ○ 🙁

How I feel today about my activities

○ 🙂   ○ 😐   ○ 🙁

Mark the pain zones

Time Started:
Time Ended:
Total Duration:

Type of pain: ☐ Tingling
☐ Shooting ☐ Throbbing
☐ Sharp ☐ Aching ☐ Swelling
☐ Burning ☐ Numbness
☐ Cramping ☐ Stiffness ☐ Dull
☐ Other: ―――――――

Front Right Back Left

Pain Scale: 1 2 3 4 5 6 7 8 9 10

SYMPTOMS

	PAIN	FATIGUE	ANXIETY	MOOD
AM	/10	/10	/10	/10
PM	/10	/10	/10	/10

TAKEN TODAY

NOTE OF THE DAY

SOMETHING TO MAKE TOMORROW BETTER:

Today's Date: _____

SLEEP _____
_____

BREAKFAST
_____
_____
_____
_____
_____

LUNCH
_____
_____
_____
_____
_____

DINNER
_____
_____
_____
_____
_____

SNACKS
_____   _____   _____
_____   _____   _____

WATER 🥤🥤🥤🥤🥤🥤🥤🥤🥤🥤🥤🥤   TOTAL: _____

ACTIVITIES
_____
_____
_____

How I feel today about my food

○ 🙂   ○ 😐   ○ ☹️

How I feel today about my activities

○ 🙂   ○ 😐   ○ ☹️

Mark the pain zones

Front   Right   Back   Left

Time Started:
Time Ended:
Total Duration:

Type of pain:
- ☐ Tingling
- ☐ Shooting ☐ Throbbing
- ☐ Sharp ☐ Aching ☐ Swelling
- ☐ Burning ☐ Numbness
- ☐ Cramping ☐ Stiffness ☐ Dull
- ☐ Other: _____

Pain Scale: 1 2 3 4 5 6 7 8 9 10

SYMPTOMS

_____   _____   _____
_____   _____   _____
_____   _____   _____

	PAIN	FATIGUE	ANXIETY	MOOD
AM	/10	/10	/10	/10
PM	/10	/10	/10	/10

TAKEN TODAY

_____   _____   _____
_____   _____   _____
_____   _____   _____

NOTE OF THE DAY

_____
_____
_____

SOMETHING TO MAKE TOMORROW BETTER:

_____
_____
_____

Today's Date : _____

SLEEP _____

BREAKFAST **LUNCH** **DINNER**

SNACKS

WATER 🥛🥛🥛🥛🥛🥛🥛🥛🥛🥛🥛🥛

TOTAL: _____

ACTIVITIES

How I feel today about my food

○ 🙂   ○ 😐   ○ 🙁

How I feel today about my activities

○ 🙂   ○ 😐   ○ 🙁

Mark the pain zones

Front Right Back Left

Time Started:
Time Ended:
Total Duration:

Type of pain: ☐ Tingling
☐ Shooting ☐ Throbbing
☐ Sharp ☐ Aching ☐ Swelling
☐ Burning ☐ Numbness
☐ Cramping ☐ Stiffness ☐ Du

☐ Other: ―――――――

Pain Scale: 1 2 3 4 5 6 7 8 9 10

SYMPTOMS

	PAIN	FATIGUE	ANXIETY	MOOD
AM	/10	/10	/10	/10
PM	/10	/10	/10	/10

TAKEN TODAY

NOTE OF THE DAY

SOMETHING TO MAKE TOMORROW BETTER:

Today's Date: _____

SLEEP
_____
_____

BREAKFAST
_____
_____
_____
_____
_____

LUNCH
_____
_____
_____
_____
_____

DINNER
_____
_____
_____
_____
_____

SNACKS
_____ _____ _____
_____ _____ _____

WATER
🥤🥤🥤🥤🥤🥤🥤🥤🥤🥤🥤

TOTAL: _____

ACTIVITIES
_____
_____
_____

How I feel today about my food

○ 🙂   ○ 😐   ○ 🙁

How I feel today about my activities

○ 🙂   ○ 😐   ○ 🙁

Mark the pain zones

Front Right Back Left

Time Started:
Time Ended:
Total Duration:

Type of pain: ☐ Tingling
☐ Shooting ☐ Throbbing
☐ Sharp ☐ Aching ☐ Swelling
☐ Burning ☐ Numbness
☐ Cramping ☐ Stiffness ☐ Dull
☐ Other: ─────────

Pain Scale: 1 2 3 4 5 6 7 8 9 10

SYMPTOMS

	PAIN	FATIGUE	ANXIETY	MOOD
AM	/10	/10	/10	/10
PM	/10	/10	/10	/10

TAKEN TODAY

NOTE OF THE DAY

SOMETHING TO MAKE TOMORROW BETTER:

Today's Date : _____

SLEEP _____
_____

BREAKFAST   **LUNCH**   **DINNER**
_____   _____   _____
_____   _____   _____
_____   _____   _____
_____   _____   _____

SNACKS
_____   _____   _____
_____   _____   _____

WATER 🍺 🍺 🍺 🍺 🍺 🍺 🍺 🍺 🍺 🍺 🍺 🍺
TOTAL: _____

ACTIVITIES
_____
_____
_____
_____

How I feel today about my food

  o 🙂   o 😐   o 🙁

How I feel today about my activities

  o 🙂   o 😐   o 🙁

Mark the pain zones

Front Right Back Left

Time Started:
Time Ended:
Total Duration:

Type of pain: ☐ Tingling
☐ Shooting ☐ Throbbing
☐ Sharp ☐ Aching ☐ Swelling
☐ Burning ☐ Numbness
☐ Cramping ☐ Stiffness ☐ Dull
☐ Other: ─────────

Pain Scale: 1 2 3 4 5 6 7 8 9 10

SYMPTOMS

_____ _____ _____
_____ _____ _____
_____ _____ _____

	PAIN	FATIGUE	ANXIETY	MOOD
AM	/10	/10	/10	/10
PM	/10	/10	/10	/10

TAKEN TODAY

_____ _____ _____
_____ _____ _____
_____ _____ _____

NOTE OF THE DAY

_____
_____
_____

SOMETHING TO MAKE TOMORROW BETTER:

_____
_____
_____

I am Strong because I'm Still Here

Today's Date : _____

SLEEP _____
     _____

BREAKFAST   LUNCH   DINNER
_____   _____   _____
_____   _____   _____
_____   _____   _____
_____   _____   _____
_____   _____   _____

SNACKS
_____   _____   _____
_____   _____   _____
_____   _____   _____

WATER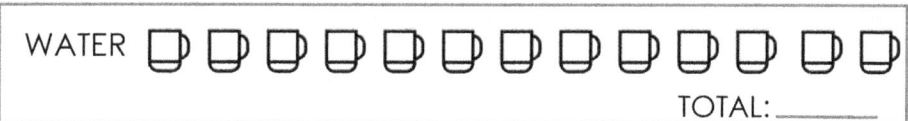
                                              TOTAL: _____

ACTIVITIES
_____
_____
_____
_____

How I feel today about my food

○    ○   ○

How I feel today about my activities

○   ○   ○

Mark the pain zones

Front Right Back Left

Time Started:
Time Ended:
Total Duration:

Type of pain: ☐ Tingling
☐ Shooting ☐ Throbbing
☐ Sharp ☐ Aching ☐ Swelling
☐ Burning ☐ Numbness
☐ Cramping ☐ Stiffness ☐ Dull
☐ Other: ―――――――

Pain Scale: 1 2 3 4 5 6 7 8 9 10

SYMPTOMS

_____ _____ _____
_____ _____ _____
_____ _____ _____

	PAIN	FATIGUE	ANXIETY	MOOD
AM	/10	/10	/10	/10
PM	/10	/10	/10	/10

TAKEN TODAY

_____ _____ _____
_____ _____ _____
_____ _____ _____

NOTE OF THE DAY

_____
_____
_____

SOMETHING TO MAKE TOMORROW BETTER:

_____
_____
_____

Today's Date : _____

SLEEP _____
_____

BREAKFAST   **LUNCH**   **DINNER**
_____   _____   _____
_____   _____   _____
_____   _____   _____
_____   _____   _____

SNACKS
_____   _____   _____
_____   _____   _____
_____   _____   _____

WATER 🥛🥛🥛🥛🥛🥛🥛🥛🥛🥛🥛🥛
TOTAL: _____

ACTIVITIES
_____
_____
_____
_____

How I feel today about my food

○ 🙂   ○ 😐   ○ ☹️

How I feel today about my activities

○ 🙂   ○ 😐   ○ ☹️

Mark the pain zones

Front   Right   Back   Left

Time Started:
Time Ended:
Total Duration:

Type of pain: ☐ Tingling
☐ Shooting   ☐ Throbbing
☐ Sharp ☐ Aching ☐ Swelling
☐ Burning   ☐ Numbness
☐ Cramping ☐ Stiffness ☐ Dull
☐ Other: ───────────

Pain Scale: 1 2 3 4 5 6 7 8 9 10

SYMPTOMS

	PAIN	FATIGUE	ANXIETY	MOOD
AM	/10	/10	/10	/10
PM	/10	/10	/10	/10

TAKEN TODAY

NOTE OF THE DAY

SOMETHING TO MAKE TOMORROW BETTER:

Today's Date : _____

SLEEP _____
_____

BREAKFAST
_____
_____
_____
_____
_____

LUNCH
_____
_____
_____
_____
_____

DINNER
_____
_____
_____
_____
_____

SNACKS
_____
_____
_____

_____
_____
_____

_____
_____
_____

WATER 🍺🍺🍺🍺🍺🍺🍺🍺🍺🍺🍺🍺

TOTAL: _____

ACTIVITIES
_____
_____
_____
_____

How I feel today about my food

○ 🙂   ○ 😐   ○ 🙁

How I feel today about my activities

○ 🙂   ○ 😐   ○ 🙁

Mark the pain zones

Front Right Back Left

Time Started:
Time Ended:
Total Duration:

Type of pain: ☐ Tingling
☐ Shooting ☐ Throbbing
☐ Sharp ☐ Aching ☐ Swelling
☐ Burning ☐ Numbness
☐ Cramping ☐ Stiffness ☐ Du
☐ Other: ─────────

Pain Scale: 1 2 3 4 5 6 7 8 9 10

SYMPTOMS

	PAIN	FATIGUE	ANXIETY	MOOD
AM	/10	/10	/10	/10
PM	/10	/10	/10	/10

TAKEN TODAY

NOTE OF THE DAY

SOMETHING TO MAKE TOMORROW BETTER:

Today's Date : _____

SLEEP _____
     _____

BREAKFAST   LUNCH   DINNER
_____   _____   _____
_____   _____   _____
_____   _____   _____
_____   _____   _____
_____   _____   _____

SNACKS
_____   _____   _____
_____   _____   _____
_____   _____   _____

WATER 🥤🥤🥤🥤🥤🥤🥤🥤🥤🥤
                              TOTAL: _____

ACTIVITIES
_____
_____
_____

How I feel today about my food

   ○ 😊   ○ 😐   ○ ☹️

How I feel today about my activities

   ○ 😊   ○ 😐   ○ ☹️

Mark the pain zones

Front   Right   Back   Left

Time Started:
Time Ended:
Total Duration:

Type of pain: ☐ Tingling
☐ Shooting ☐ Throbbing
☐ Sharp ☐ Aching ☐ Swelling
☐ Burning ☐ Numbness
☐ Cramping ☐ Stiffness ☐ Dull
☐ Other: ─────────

Pain Scale: 1 2 3 4 5 6 7 8 9 10

SYMPTOMS

_____ _____ _____
_____ _____ _____
_____ _____ _____

	PAIN	FATIGUE	ANXIETY	MOOD
AM	/10	/10	/10	/10
PM	/10	/10	/10	/10

TAKEN TODAY

_____ _____ _____
_____ _____ _____
_____ _____ _____

NOTE OF THE DAY

_____
_____
_____

SOMETHING TO MAKE TOMORROW BETTER:

_____
_____
_____

Today's Date : _____

SLEEP _____
_____

BREAKFAST
_____
_____
_____
_____
_____

LUNCH
_____
_____
_____
_____
_____

DINNER
_____
_____
_____
_____
_____

SNACKS
_____
_____
_____

_____
_____
_____

_____
_____
_____

WATER 🍺 🍺 🍺 🍺 🍺 🍺 🍺 🍺 🍺 🍺 🍺 🍺

TOTAL: _____

ACTIVITIES
_____
_____
_____
_____

How I feel today about my food

○ 🙂   ○ 😐   ○ 🙁

How I feel today about my activities

○ 🙂   ○ 😐   ○ 🙁

Mark the pain zones

Front   Right   Back   Left

Time Started:
Time Ended:
Total Duration:

Type of pain: ☐ Tingling
☐ Shooting ☐ Throbbing
☐ Sharp ☐ Aching ☐ Swelling
☐ Burning ☐ Numbness
☐ Cramping ☐ Stiffness ☐ Dull
☐ Other: ─────────

Pain Scale: 1 2 3 4 5 6 7 8 9 10

SYMPTOMS

	PAIN	FATIGUE	ANXIETY	MOOD
AM	/10	/10	/10	/10
PM	/10	/10	/10	/10

TAKEN TODAY

NOTE OF THE DAY

SOMETHING TO MAKE TOMORROW BETTER:

Today's Date : _____

SLEEP _____
_____

BREAKFAST
_____
_____
_____
_____
_____

LUNCH
_____
_____
_____
_____
_____

DINNER
_____
_____
_____
_____
_____

SNACKS
_____
_____
_____

_____
_____
_____

_____
_____
_____

WATER 🥛🥛🥛🥛🥛🥛🥛🥛🥛🥛🥛🥛

TOTAL: _____

ACTIVITIES
_____
_____
_____
_____

How I feel today about my food

○ 🙂   ○ 😐   ○ 🙁

How I feel today about my activities

○ 🙂   ○ 😐   ○ 🙁

Mark the pain zones

Front Right Back Left

Time Started:
Time Ended:
Total Duration:

Type of pain: ☐ Tingling
☐ Shooting ☐ Throbbing
☐ Sharp ☐ Aching ☐ Swelling
☐ Burning ☐ Numbness
☐ Cramping ☐ Stiffness ☐ Du
☐ Other: ─────────

Pain Scale: 1 2 3 4 5 6 7 8 9 10

SYMPTOMS

_____ _____ _____
_____ _____ _____
_____ _____ _____

	PAIN	FATIGUE	ANXIETY	MOOD
AM	/10	/10	/10	/10
PM	/10	/10	/10	/10

TAKEN TODAY

_____ _____ _____
_____ _____ _____
_____ _____ _____

NOTE OF THE DAY

_____
_____
_____

SOMETHING TO MAKE TOMORROW BETTER:

_____
_____
_____

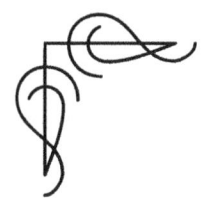
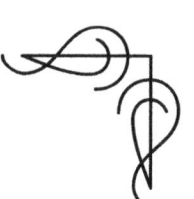

Doctors/Clinic appointments

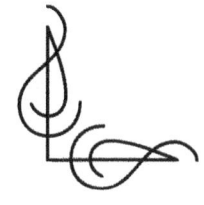
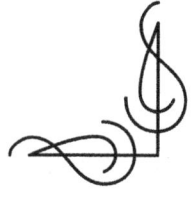

Date	Time	With	Reason

NOTES/RESULT

Date	Time	With	Reason

NOTES/RESULT

Date	Time	With	Reason

NOTES/RESULT

Date	Time	With	Reason

NOTES/RESULT

_____
_____
_____
_____
_____

Date	Time	With	Reason

NOTES/RESULT

_____
_____
_____
_____
_____

Date	Time	With	Reason

NOTES/RESULT

_____
_____
_____
_____
_____

Date	Time	With	Reason

NOTES/RESULT

Date	Time	With	Reason

NOTES/RESULT

Date	Time	With	Reason

NOTES/RESULT

Date	Time	With	Reason

NOTES/RESULT

Date	Time	With	Reason

NOTES/RESULT

Date	Time	With	Reason

NOTES/RESULT

Date	Time	With	Reason

NOTES/RESULT

_____
_____
_____
_____
_____

Date	Time	With	Reason

NOTES/RESULT

_____
_____
_____
_____
_____

Date	Time	With	Reason

NOTES/RESULT

_____
_____
_____
_____
_____

Date	Time	With	Reason

NOTES/RESULT

Date	Time	With	Reason

NOTES/RESULT

Date	Time	With	Reason

NOTES/RESULT

And don't forget:

YOU ARE VALUABLE
JUST BECAUSE YOU EXIST.
NOT BECAUSE OF WHAT YOU DO
OR WHAT YOU HAVE DONE,
BUT SIMPLY BECAUSE
YOU ARE.

never give up

Made in the USA
Las Vegas, NV
20 January 2022